I0428649

Printed in the United States of America

ISBN 978-1502767097

First Printing, 2014

CONTENTS

Breakfast Is A Must.. 4

Eat More Filling Food.................................... 7

Meal Planning... 10

Build Lean Muscle.. 14

Track Progress And Develop Reward System.............. 17

Coping With Temptation.................................. 21

Motivation.. 24

Eliminate Unnecessary Beverages....................... 27

Late Night Eating.. 31

Stress Rest And Sleep.................................... 34

Cardiovascular Exercise.................................. 38

Get Creative.. 42

Maintenance Is A Way Of Life........................... 47

Weight loss and fitness is a common goal for many people. The reason most people struggle in this area is because they fail to embrace its natural and scientific simplicity. No diet is ever going to truly result in you keeping weight off in the long run and completing lifetime fitness objectives. In order to do so, you will have to become somewhat educated and smarter with your personal choices.

Within this book's pages you'll learn the Importance of: Eating Breakfast, Eating More Filling Foods, Planning Your Meals, Building Lean Muscles, Tracking Your Progress, Coping with Temptation, Dealing with Stress, Cardiovascular Exercise and So Much More!

This book is written in a clear cut and to the point fashion in order to accommodate people of all ages, sizes, weights and fitness levels. It carries a tone of pure simplicity that might be deemed TOO SIMPLE. But, the reason most people struggle in this area of life is because they're not mindful of the simplicity of it all.

Permanent weight loss and fitness requires a consistent lifestyle cycle of pursuing, maintaining and expanding upon your health and fitness goals.

The twelve (12) powerful principles shared in this book can be incorporated into your daily life so that you can Take Back Your Body for good.

Breakfast Is A Must

Would you ever get into your vehicle to drive somewhere without any gas? Of course you wouldn't, and that is no way to start your day either. For sure, the fried potatoes, grits and gravy and buttermilk biscuits should not be your daily breakfast staples, but that doesn't mean you should forget breakfast. Yogurt, fruit, and oatmeal are a few healthy options.

Forget breakfast and everything else you do concerning your weight loss and fitness goals is going to suffer. That is why developing a habit of eating a healthy breakfast each day is the first step. For beverages, choose from milk, healthy all-natural juices, and water. Not that you absolutely have to give up coffee, but it's certainly worth the contemplation if you're able.

People often mistakenly think that skipping breakfast because they are not hungry is going to help them lose weight faster. Instead, they are facilitating a cycle in which their body is always behind the eight ball. If you're not sold yet, then understand that it is common knowledge that breakfast jump starts your metabolism for the day and also, gets the digestive processes flowing.

Imagine you skip breakfast. Can you see yourself eating more for lunch and dinner? Another thing that often occurs when a person skips breakfast is the indulgence in high calorie snacks. Starting off with a proper breakfast can alter your mood, provide your body with fuel, and help you better navigate your way through daily snacks, meals and food choices in general.

Eating a healthy breakfast is going to play a huge part in watching your portions throughout the day and eating smaller, more frequent meals. You will make better food choices overall as well because you will be working to help naturally suppress your appetite and keep any food binges or unhealthy choices at bay.

A healthy breakfast can also help you lower your cholesterol levels, which is a focus of many people, especially as you age. A healthy breakfast gets your brain going for the day and provides you with more strength, endurance, energy and improved concentration and performance according to medical professionals.

Do you have children? This is a good time to get you started thinking about changes to their daily lifestyles, as well. You want to provide them with a solid background regarding health and fitness, and breakfast has everything to do with a healthy foundation and start to their day. In fact, medical professionals say that breakfast is especially important for children because it helps improve their classroom performance and participation in other activities, focus, hand-eye coordination, and problem-solving skills.

EAT MORE FILLING FOODS

It is a common joke that when eating Chinese food, a person is hungry a couple hours later. This is not the desired outcome. Studies have shown that people are able to lose weight and keep that weight off much easier when they are knowledgeable about and pursue eating more filling foods. Naturally, these need to be healthy food choices as well.

Women especially can have a harder time dropping pounds and toning their bodies. For everyone, eating more filling foods is a step that, when implemented, can be a game changer. This can help you with calorie counting, and it can help you avoid eating unhealthy snacks during time crunches.

Look for healthy foods that are high in fiber, which are not only going to be more filling but also aid your body's digestive process. Think lean proteins, whole grains and fruits and vegetables. You can see why oatmeal is a great breakfast choice now, as this can be a low-calorie filling breakfast that gets you to your next meal time. A baked potato is a healthy and filling option for lunch or as a side for dinner. Potatoes are filling, but just be sure you use healthy toppings!

Healthy soups are always hearty choices, such as bean or split-pea soup. Eggs, yogurt, apples and popcorn are also healthy and filling options. Perhaps you've seen the busy worker carrying around an apple. Many people don't realize that popcorn can be a nice healthy and filling snack. Of course, you can't eat the theater popcorn loaded with fake butter and expect it to fit into your dietary regimen!

When you're eating those raw vegetables for snacks, make sure you don't leave out the dip, albeit a healthy dip. You can use different hummus flavors as dip or whatever you like, but experts say this is necessary to help the vegetables be more filling. As long as you're adding something healthy, you're fine.

When choosing high-fiber and filling foods; you definitely want to take a look at your bean and legume options. Beans, while very good for you and filing, can also add up calories quite quickly, so you want to eat them in small portions or add them to other dishes.

Don't forget about nuts! There are so many types of delicious nuts. You can use them in other recipes as well. Enjoying a small bag of almonds not only is filling and works as a natural appetite suppressant, but also provides many other health benefits. Nuts are full of protein, and they are a top choice for that intermediate snack.

Nuts also contain healthy fats, which are an essential part of your diet. You need these fats, and you're working on eliminating other unhealthy fats. Your serving size should be kept to about 12 nuts, or you can choose to make a dish with them, such as unique orange-scented green beans with toasted almonds. Pistachios and pecans are two other tasty choices when looking at nuts for snacks or to use in your kitchen creations.

MEAL PLANNING

Your overall weight loss and fitness plan is going to benefit immensely from planning out your meals. No doubt life these days continues to move at an even quicker pace, and it's easy to get caught up in all the hustle and bustle, sacrificing your diet. Skipping breakfast has already been discussed. Don't find yourself hitting the drive-thru when on lunch break or to hurriedly trying to throw together dinner for the kids.

Start with gathering healthy recipes. Plan out what meals you want to cook for each day, and write all the ingredients you need down on a grocery list. Don't forget to add the healthy snacks you need for rushed times or for in between meals. If you're able to do so, you can actually prepare and cook your meals ahead of time so that you're not stuck cooking each day.

How you handle meal preparation and planning is up to you. But it is definitely a key to ensuring you don't get caught sacrificing your dietary needs and throwing whatever you can find down the chute into your stomach.

Perhaps for one day, you have purchased all the ingredients to make a healthy stir fry with lean meat, rice and vegetables. For another dinner, you might plan to prepare a family-sized grilled chicken Caesar salad. You're going to have to put in the time and preparation, but you're going to actually find it eliminates the stress concerning food choices and helps motivate you towards your goals. You will feel much more control over your daily meals.

Food these days is quite expensive, and buying all those ingredients can add up. That is why two simple recipes were mentioned in the previous paragraph. Always search out simple and delicious recipes to save money and use coupons. There are also food planner apps available that can further assist you with keeping up with planning out your meals.

When planning out your meals ahead of time, you are also able to save money. It has been noted many times that eating healthy can actually cost a person money;

however, this truly depends on the approach. There are all kinds of ways to cut corners as already mentioned, and you're going to preventing impulsive dinner buying as well. Not only that, but you're going to better be able to control portions.

One thing you must really think about when planning out your meals is waste. For instance, if you're cooking your meals ahead of time, you want to have them stored properly. Think ahead of time about what space you have, in your cupboards, refrigerator and freezer. This all gets easier with time, but as you get started, really pay attention to what you're doing. The last thing you want is to end up throwing money down the drain because food spoils.

If you have children, you want to not only involve them in the meal planning at home, but also ensure that they are eating healthy when at school. Kids are going to want their pizza, cake and ice cream, especially at special occasions. Face it; special occasions happen for kids quite often! Still, you want to be teaching them the healthy habits that you're including in your life.

Now, after you finish this book and have all the necessary tools to develop a long-lasting lifestyle weight loss and fitness plan, you are challenged to do something immediately. You are challenged to go to the kitchen and begin the overhaul. You're going to learn about different things that might surprisingly keep certain things in your kitchen, but you are undoubtedly going to make several changes. Furthermore, you're going to want to subsequently pay a visit to the grocery store and get everything else you need. It's going to be your first order of business, and you should be plenty excited to get going!

BUILD LEAN MUSCLE

One of the biggest mistakes people make when designing exercise regimens is not including lifting weights. Yes, cardiovascular exercise is very important when it comes to burning calories and trimming your physique, among other benefits; however, building lean muscle using weight lifting exercises helps increase your metabolism.

Simple science states that lean muscle has a higher metabolism than does fat. Therefore, you can see how building lean muscle can help to jump-start your metabolism. This doesn't mean you have to build big muscles; instead, you're going to consistently include muscle building exercises in your fitness regimen two to three days a week for 30 minutes. Make sure you continue to evaluate your muscle building routine so that you keep challenging yourself.

You can incorporate weight lifting into your fitness and exercise regimen without being a bodybuilder as mentioned. Whether you join a gym, take classes or use home equipment or free weights is up to you. Push yourself to complete reps, trying for one every two seconds. Furthermore, aim for muscle fatigue, and allow yourself one minute of rest in between reps.

The best lean muscle exercises can also be compound exercises. Pushups top the list, and no equipment is even required to perform this exercise. Kettle bell workouts, TRX bands and weight lifting on your tip toes are also good options. Have you heard of Burpees? Burpees are a compound step by step exercise that incorporates and combines core work, jumping, squatting and pushups all in one exercise.

Now, building lean muscle is not just about muscle building exercises. This is where more of your eating plan is also going to come together. One food that you can eat to help you build muscle is brown rice, which provides you with extra energy as a whole-grain food that digests slowly. Brown rice can also work to help you boost your GH or growth hormone levels naturally.

Beets are another food that can help you build lean muscle, as well as oranges, cantaloupe and cottage cheese. Eggs and apples were previously mentioned in a different chapter, and they make the list here as well. Spinach, quinoa and organic milk are also good choices.

One more food that should be added to your list is ground beef. Now, this seems counter-intuitive since you should definitely be limiting your intake of red meat. However, eating a couple servings of red meat each week is actually balanced and fits right in with a healthy lifestyle and building lean muscle. The key here is balance.

TRACK PROGRESS AND DEVELOP REWARD SYSTEM

You are already going to be planning your meals and scheduling an exercise regimen. As results are realized, you and others are going to be taking notice. Wouldn't you like to have a record of where you've been? Wouldn't keeping track of your progress be motivating?

For starters, you're going to weigh yourself daily. Now, you might be thinking that everything you've read so far is spot on, but how can this be helpful? Did you know that studies actually prove and show that people who weigh themselves daily are twice as likely to keep off weight that they have lost? That statistic alone should be enough to get you hopping on the scale each day.

You don't have to think of it as a hassle; instead, weigh yourself in the morning as you are getting ready for the day. If you have a lot of weight to lose and find daily weigh-ins a little frustrating at the beginning, use this for motivation. These weigh-ins are going to become increasingly important as you move closer to the maintenance phase.

Now you might be thinking okay that's enough recording and planning. If this is what you're thinking, then you should be reminded that most of the planning mentioned in earlier chapters is actually going to simplify your life and reduce stress. That is the result of organization. So, as you record your weight daily, you have a little time to record your thoughts. On top of recording your thoughts, you need to be counting calories consumed and calories burned. If you're planning your meals, this should be pretty simple as you can take a look at everything ahead of time. For sure, one key aspect of losing weight will always be burning more calories than you consume daily.

Counting calories is not just about weight loss; it's going to be used in the maintenance phase as well. Furthermore, as you plan out your exercise regimen, leave a spot for recording calories burned. While all of this may seem a bit complicated at first, it gets easier with time. You are going to familiarize yourself with calories burned for certain exercises.

You are also going to familiarize yourself with calorie counts for food items. This can be particularly helpful when it comes to future food choices as well. For example a regular-sized red apple with the skin is 116 calories. Imagine going through your day and having this kind of knowledge so that you can keep your calorie counting in range. Sure, you will be planning your meals, but plans don't always work out. This way you have a backup plan, the knowledge of nutritious food choices to make quick and healthy decisions.

Finally, develop a reward system, in which you give yourself rewards as you reach certain goals. These don't have to be weight loss goals. They can be fitness goals or end-of-the-week rewards. Try to think of rewards that are not food-related so that you stay on track; however, food-related rewards are going to be discussed in a later chapter.

What are some ideas for rewards? Maybe as you notice a change in clothing size, you can go buy yourself a new outfit. Treat yourself to an afternoon at a health spa, or enjoy an amusement park trip with the family. Depending on your circumstances and what you enjoy, you certainly can come up with personal rewards. The expensive rewards can be saved for major milestones, and the smaller rewards can be for your weekly achievements.

COPING WITH TEMPTATION

It is no secret that dealing with cravings and sacrificing favorite foods is a huge part of why people are unsuccessful when dieting. Of course, you're not on a diet. You're making a lifestyle change that is going to help you take back your body through weight loss and fitness. Still, how can you deal with those cravings? What can you do to resist temptation?

Obviously, the answer is not going to be that you give into temptation every time. However, you also should not be completely depriving yourself of foods you enjoy and special treats. A good rule of thumb is to allow yourself one cheat each week. This is where you enjoy a food choice you are craving. This doesn't mean you overindulge; instead, you simply allow yourself a small portion. This enables you to have better willpower when it comes to resisting your cravings throughout the rest of the week.

Now, when it comes to temptation coping outside of your once a week indulgence; think about substitutes. For example, enjoying a nice healthy yet tasty and delicious cup of Greek yogurt is much better than eating ice cream. Yogurt was also mentioned in a previous chapter concerning lean muscle building foods, and it is also a great in-between meals snack.

While you have been urged to cheat once a week, you must be certain that you stick to this plan. Obviously, too many cheats result in derailed weight loss efforts. Furthermore, as you expand your knowledge about food substitutes and your body adjusts to healthier eating, temptation coping will become easier for you.

Since you're going to be counting calories, you can always make adjustments throughout your day to your daily plan. You're going to find this happening more often than you think. Perhaps you are at work and there are surprise goodies in the break room. Go with the flow and indulge a little, and then make your calculated deductions for later.

The only rule of thumb is not to sacrifice any meals or snacks, as well as your completion of a well-balanced daily diet. If you find yourself doing this to make the calorie count, then you're indulging a little too much. Mistakes can be made and calculations can cut it close. Remember that you can always offset calories consumed with calories burned and you will win if you give it your best effort.

MOTIVATION

Motivation to some degree has already been discussed; however, you need a definitive plan for motivation. For starters, imagine watching a weight loss program. What are you going to see? For sure, you're going to be shown before and after photos. Document your efforts not only with a before photo, but also with periodic photos to show progress.

Instead of just weighing yourself daily, take measurements from time to time. It is common knowledge that you're going to be losing inches and sometimes, those inches drop without any weight loss.

Leave positive notes for yourself. No doubt, each day is a new day. Imagine waking up in the morning. You're not always going to necessarily quickly recall everything that you need to get going; however, a positive note from the night before left on the fridge might help do the trick. Or, you can leave yourself a note in your journal and leave your journal in the bathroom for you to find as you're getting ready in the morning.

Another very motivating aspect of weight loss is not to go it alone. If you're going to lose weight and keep it off, you must want it for yourself; however, that doesn't mean you don't need the support of others. There are many ways you can make this happen.

First, you can ask family and friends to join you on your workouts. This can also give you fresh ideas. For example, you might ask someone to walk in the park with you that would rather play tennis. Perhaps you have never played tennis, and you decide to play once a week with this person. When people join you during your workouts, this helps keep you going, and of course it helps the other person, too.

Another way you can find support regarding your weight loss efforts is through joining weight loss support groups. There is most certainly going to be one meeting in your area. You can even start your own if you have enough people motivated to lose weight. Perhaps your immediate family is engaged in your health and fitness lifestyle changes and wants to join in the fun.

Some of the weight loss support groups in your area might be for a specific dietary plan, such as Weight Watchers. This is just an example, but Weight Watchers is essentially calorie counting using their point system, and the goals and objectives fall in line with everything you're learning and going to be implementing from this book. These groups generally meet once a week, and this can be a very constructive way to spend your time sharing with others and motivating yourself to continue on the right path.

Perhaps you can start a weight loss group or competition at work. This can be a great way to get everyone else motivated on top of giving yourself the drive that you need. Friendly competitions are fun, and there are going to be extra rewards and incentives. You can start a small cash pool with friends, or you can get HR to hold a full-blown weight loss competition for anyone who would like to join.

ELIMINATE UNNECESSARY BEVERAGES

It is possible to shed a few pounds just by eliminating sodas from your daily diet and drinking an adequate amount of water daily. Of course, you're not looking to lose a few pounds; instead, you're changing your life. Still, it's time to realize just how much the liquid part of your diet has to do with your success.

Aside from the obvious of drinking more water and staying away from sodas, there are many other ideas to implement to make the liquid part of your diet well-rounded. What types of juices do you like? There is orange juice, grape juice, apple juice, and there are even fruit and vegetable fusion juices available. Did you know that one glass of orange juice has 60 percent of the vitamin C your body needs daily?

Have you heard of green tea? Originating in China, this beverage has been the subject of many medical and scientific studies in recent years. As a matter of fact, studies have shown that green tea induces thermo genesis by way of polyphenols and caffeine. This helps to increase your body's metabolism by as much as four percent. Green tea also has more flavonoids in comparison to other beverages, and these flavonoids are responsible for anticarcinogenic and antioxidative functions.

If you're still finding it rather boring trying to stay away from sodas, all you have to do is get a little creative. Try out fruit smoothies using whole fruit, milk and ice. You can even have all-natural supplemental ingredients to these smoothies so that you are supplementing your daily nutrition. It is especially helpful when adding proteins to your smoothies, as people's diets are often protein deficient. Your diet should not be protein deficient, however, because you have already read the chapter about building lean muscle!

Some ingredients that you can add to smoothies are kale, chia seeds, goji berries, camu-camu, cacao powder, maca, wheat grass, coconut oil, avocados, and protein powders.

Chia seeds, for instance, are an extra source of protein, giving you added energy, and they also are touted as having many other health benefits. The chia seeds also help to thicken your smoothie.

Other beverages that you can indulge in that make the cut are mint tea and other herbal teas, hot chocolate, and soy milk. Do not sell yourself short when thinking about fruit juices because there are so many different combinations. Remember the smoothies, and you can also make low-fat ice cream or frozen yogurt shakes. As well, soy milk is mentioned as a milk substitution and when drinking regular milk, it is best to go with one percent or reduced fat.

When it comes to sodas, many people find them extremely difficult to give up, just like with coffee for others. Therefore, people tend to use diet coke and other zero or low calorie soda options as an excuse. If you absolutely must indulge in your diet sodas; however, understand that while they may not mess up your calorie count, they are not specifically helping you facilitate your weight loss and health goals. They are very acidic and the unnatural ingredients contained in them have associated with other known issues, as well.

The unnatural ingredients in soda are a good segway for a special point in the planning process that does not have its own chapter. You certainly want to be seeking out all-natural ingredients for your other beverage and food choices as well. You are going to notice more and more of these advertisements for foods that while they sound tasty, are just loaded with unnecessary sugars and all kinds of artificial ingredients and preservatives. As you get used to eating and living differently, these unhealthy choices will begin to look less and less appealing.

LATE NIGHT EATING

This topic has been of major debate over the years, with many professionals touting don't eat after 8 p.m. and many other professionals saying that this is not healthy, attributing it to a fast. Furthermore, they say that it doesn't actually help you lose weight or fall in line with a healthy lifestyle. This book is going to take the stance that a healthy well-balanced dinner should be eaten no later than 8 pm; however, healthy snacking is reserved for late night eating.

Late night eating should be defined here. Considering the next chapter is about sleep and rest, this does not mean you're going to pull out the celery sticks and peanut butter at two in the morning. No, think more along the lines of how the book mentioned already that you should be eating smaller more frequent meals each day. This equates to one healthy snack after dinner; however, do not eat this snack within the hour before you go to bed.

Eating right before you go to bed can greatly affect your digestion and cause you all kinds of problems. For one, you might not be able to fall asleep. Second, you might cause yourself some stomach pain and discomfort. While medical professionals now say that eating healthy snacks right before bed doesn't affect your weight loss efforts, the aforementioned symptoms are enough to convince most people not to eat during the hour before bedtime.

So what are some good late night snacks? You're definitely already stocking up on healthy foods and you should have quite the selection available to you. To give you some ideas, why not try spinach and artichoke grilled cheese or a red roasted pepper dip or a healthy vegetarian lo mien?

The three dishes in the previous paragraph were meant to help get your creative juices flowing when it comes to not only thinking up healthy late night snacks, but also when planning out your other meals and snacks as mentioned in the other chapter. Since you are planning ahead of time, you are going to be able to look up delicious and unique recipes like those, and you will have bought the ingredients ahead of time to make them. When you're concocting creative dishes like that, you're not going to miss the unhealthy alternatives any longer.

Perhaps you have a sweet tooth craving at night and this is when you like to enjoy a nice dessert. There are so many different ways that you can enjoy many of the nice treats you may not think you could eat, such as milkshakes, cookies, brownies and more. All the sudden those claims that you can eat what you want and still lose weight don't sound too far from the truth; however, these are modified and substitute recipes, and you're still going to be counting your calories. Still, you're in for some good late night treats!

You can also think of late night sweet treats as daily rewards. You have made it to the end of your day, and this is also a good time to record your progress and thoughts. You're going to weigh in the morning, but the night time is when you finish counting calories consumed and burned, as well as reflect upon what else happened during the day. So how many calories are you going to reserve for that late night snack?

STRESS REST AND SLEEP

Stress, rest and sleep are so intertwined that they are going to be the focus of this chapter together. Did you know that a lack of sleep can lead to an increase in the hormone that causes you to be hungry? In fact, scientists have proven this; furthermore, it decreases the hormone that makes you feel full. Therefore, this is one solid reason that you should be getting an adequate amount of sleep daily.

Stress can cause you to lose sleep. Everyone's life is different, but you know yourself the best. What is causing you stress in your life? Perhaps you're always penny pinching to make ends meet, or maybe you're worried about a specific relationship. Perhaps you have things coming at you from all directions. In order to give your body rest and enough sleep, you must be working at reducing the stress in your life.

Stress not only can hinder or manipulate your sleep pattern, but it can also cause other issues with your body, your weight loss efforts and your fitness goals. Research also shows that a lack of sleep can lead to chaos within your fat cells, causing overeating and actual weight gain. Everything else you have read is about eating the right foods and snacking so that you're not overeating. Naturally, you don't want to work against all of this by sacrificing your daily sleep.

Everyone has a different schedule. What you consider time for bed is going to find many others awake conducting business and vice versa. Do you work during the day and sleep at night? If you follow the typical nine to five schedule, that is eight hours worth of work, which leaves you 16 hours remaining out of your day. With eight hours of sleep, you're still given a third of your day to do as you please.

The fact that life moves extremely fast these days was mentioned previously, and this can be both the cause of stress and for not allowing yourself to sleep the suggested eight hours. It makes sense on paper, but sure it's difficult. It's something everyone has to deal with, and you're just going to have to convince yourself that it's a very important part of your plan.

Working against yourself in any form is going to cancel out other positive things you're doing, and you don't want to disappoint yourself on the scale. People think that if they get more done and stay up that the sacrifice couldn't possibly be bad. They couldn't be more wrong when it comes to their health, fitness objectives and weight loss and maintenance efforts.

What you also must consider is consistency. This can be the most difficult part of getting enough sleep. One night, you might get home at nine and not be able to get to bed until after midnight. The next night, you might have a regular schedule and become tired at ten. This is just an example, but you can see how situations can fluctuate if you reflect upon your own past experiences.

All you can do is give it your best. You're going to run into extraordinary circumstances that affect many other aspect of your weight loss and fitness plan as well. You're going to make choices, such as staying out late on a weekend for a special vacation or disrupting your sleep schedule while on vacation. No plan is going to work out perfectly, but knowing what comprises a winning plan will help you stay on track as much as possible. If you fall off the wagon with your sleep consistency or any other part of your diet, put a smile on your face and keep on going. You're in this for life!

How many hours do you work each week? Often, extra work is due to financial stress, and work cutting into your personal time can itself impact your efforts to get enough sleep. People find themselves working two and three jobs, waking up again after four hours of sleep and doing it all over again. Are you a student? Students often sacrifice their sleep and health working their way through school and attending classes. Think about how you can make adjustments to your personal circumstances, so you can really see this lifestyle change take effect.

CARDIOVASCULAR EXERCISE

A previous chapter focused on exercise when it comes to your personal fitness, health and weight loss goals promoted lean muscle building. This chapter is going to focus on the cardiovascular exercise aspect of your fitness regimen. Unlike lean muscle building, where your muscle groups need rest days, you should be participating in cardiovascular exercise for at least 30 minutes each day.

The mistake that people often make not just with cardiovascular exercise, but with exercise in general, is not being creative. Creative thinking was a major focus when it came to both planning out your meals and especially late night snacks and sweet desserts. Creativity is part of the imagination process, expanding your mind, and it is a must when it comes to implementing lifestyle changes. After all, it's bad habits and daily routines combined with fast-paced lifestyles that is wreaking havoc on people's bodies.

Maybe you enjoy getting on the treadmill daily while watching your favorite television show, or perhaps you have an exercise video or a daily exercise class. Maybe you're a speed walker in the park, taking in the scenery. All of this is fine, but there are going to be days that you just don't feel like doing these things. Motivation was a chapter all by itself, and motivation as it pertains to cardiovascular exercise is ensuring you have backup plans and creative ideas.

Maybe you can't get to the gym one day, or perhaps you're out of town on vacation. Maybe you're used to playing a sport with someone on a certain day, and that person calls and cancels. For sure, if you enjoy doing a particular cardiovascular exercise daily, pursue this activity with fervor, but always try new things as well.

Want some ideas? This first one might be a little expensive, but what are you doing for your next vacation? Why not go for some cross-country skiing? Skiing itself is a great form of cardiovascular exercise, and you can also choose to snowboard. Maybe you're lucky enough to live in such an environment. If not, why not go for a swim, or maybe you would like to bike around town.

Bicycling is even better if you live in rural areas. Surely, you can already see that a key to being creative when it comes to cardiovascular exercise is taking advantage of the environment in which you live. Another rule of thumb is to take advantage of the outdoors as often as possible. Again, daily running on the treadmill watching television is not a bad thing; however, at least try to shake things up from time to time with a little excitement outside. This also opens you up to more social possibilities with exercise, which was also mentioned when it comes to motivation.

Reducing stress is a focus, so why not let it all out while learning the sport of kickboxing? Whatever you choose to do, you're going to have to assess your personal fitness level and know your limits. When in doubt, you should always consult your family doctor.

Some people are limited as to the space they have to work out. Many times, you might seek out other establishments or take things outdoors; however, you need options for when you're in a time crunch and stuck with the small space. Why not buy a stair stepper? It beats fitting a treadmill or other piece of fitness equipment within your domicile. The use of certain fitness videos will work for smaller spaces; however, another option is purchasing a medicine ball to do cardiovascular exercise at home.

If the floor within your home is sturdy, and you don't live on a floor directly above someone, you can always run or jog in place. The point being here is to get the job done. Whether you have limited space or all the space in the world and a personal trainer, you're going to have those days where you need creative options for various reasons, such as being displaced for the day or out of time or otherwise occupied.

GET CREATIVE!

You asked for it, and you got it! Okay, well you didn't ask for it, but did you really think you were going to make it out of this book without reading more about creativity? It's time to get those juices flowing with some suggestions.

Wearing a pedometer daily can help you achieve extra exercise and benefits you in other ways as well. First, it can help you with the recording of your calories burned and daily fitness. Aren't you looking to burn as many calories as you can? Well, when calculating your daily calorie burn, a pedometer can help that number go up! The reason for this is the pedometer gives you the mindset for seeking extra steps and opportunities for exercise.

Perhaps you park your vehicle in the parking space at the end of the parking lot when hit the store. You become quite familiar then how many more steps you take in just for this simple exercise. Maybe you're on your way home from visiting someone on a weekend afternoon. You spent a couple of hours sitting and talking, and the sun is out shining. All of the sudden, you see your pedometer and find yourself veering off in the direction of the park for a nice walk.

What kind of job do you have? If you're a construction worker out in the hot sun all day, then you don't have anything to worry about; however if you're working in an office, creativity is definitely going to have to come into play here. The office job must be addressed because you can find yourself sitting for long hours. Many people with office jobs tend to exercise during their lunch breaks or right after work. Some companies provide on-site gym access, and this is something you might want to check out. Even if you just hop on the exercise bike for 15 minutes, it's worth the extra effort.

People often find ways to exercise at their desk as well. If you're consistently meeting with or communicating with people, this can be difficult; however, there are ways you can exercise while sitting at your desk, making this a possibility for some people, perhaps yourself.

When planning meals, you want to make things look appealing. This means you're going to have to have to cook, and you're going to want to use whole foods. Fruits and vegetables are colorful, and doesn't a colorful plate look much more delicious? Furthermore, a lack of color often symbolizes an unhealthy meal, which means you should do the color check since you're already supposed to be preparing healthy meals.

Pack yourself some gum. There are going to be those times when you are just in between and can't seem to stick to your meal schedule. Packing different types of healthy snacks is always key, but gum is especially important. First of all, some delicious cinnamon gum is more easily kept in your pocket, and it is also less calories. Gum also works as a helpful appetite suppressant, so it can buy you some time when you're in a crunch.

Remember that chapter about sleep, stress and relaxation? A busy day at work is stressful enough. A working person devotes approximately a third of his or her life to working. Allow yourself moments to relieve stress and just relax throughout your day. Everyone needs a little peace and quiet time. Perhaps you indulge in your moment when you first get home from work. You might sit down in a comfortable chair and just let everything go. Or, maybe you take a soak in the hot tub!

Whatever you do, you need to find those moments throughout your day in which you can just relax. Naturally, this will help facilitate your regular sleep schedule. There are all kinds of ways you can achieve this goal, but again everyone's life is different. Some people live alone, and others have six children and a spouse with the same schedule! Wherever you fall in between there, think and you will come up with the solution. Even if you're just spending the last 30 minutes of your day before bed lying next to your spouse reading a book, it counts.

Are you ready to hear that television is bad for you? Certainly you're not thinking that you're going to just be told it keeps you sitting down and not exercising. Surely that is one point, but what about all of those delicious commercials you see for foods you're not supposed to be eating?

Now, remember that you're already equipped with creative recipes and substitutions, meal planning, a strong fitness regimen and more frequent meals. Still, too much television takes away time from your day and can ultimately impact many different aspects of your plan, such as adequate sleep, exercise, time spent outdoors and more.

Furthermore, group the idea of watching television consistently with the commercials that are shown and the activity of actually eating simultaneously. This can easily lead to slip-ups, especially at social gatherings. And, don't forget those birthday parties, Super Bowl Sundays and other celebrations you attend. Remember that you're supposed to allow yourself to cheat from time to time but just not overindulge. On these special occasions, you can find ways to skate by at times, or you can choose to use these as your cheat.

MAINTENANCE IS A WAY OF LIFE

The twelve steps to taking back your body have already been outlined; however, what happens when you've taken your body back? Indeed, there is always work to be done. Furthermore, losing the weight and keeping it off requires a life-long commitment and lifestyle change. This can be referred to as 'maintenance,' as the following explanation will help explain.

Say you've reached your goal weight. Your last checkup at the doctor was excellent. You feel great, and the sun is shining. Okay, in all seriousness, you already realize the lifestyle change and have achieved your goals. Even though you've lost all the weight, you're still used to counting calories and continue to count them. You work out just as vigorously, and you do everything as you normally do. There are two things to consider here.

First, how long did it take you to get there? Most likely, you've spent some time by then, but you're talking a few years or so at the most. Are you just going to keep doing the same thing for the rest of your life? No, the maintenance phase of your life is going to change through the years. You're going to get older! Your activities and dietary habits are going to change as well as what your body needs.

Second, immediately after successfully completing a weight loss goal, the maintenance phase is more easily defined as keeping the weight off and your body in shape. This is going to require balancing out your calories eaten and burned. Now, instead of not working out as much to burn all those calories, it is instead suggested that you increase the amount of calories consumed to maintain your weight. Of course, you're going to keep those food choices healthy!

From breakfast full cycle to getting enough sleep and waking up again for a healthy breakfast has been laid out for you. It is extremely important that you develop a strong plan moving forward with your weight loss and fitness goals. Not addressing any areas of an overall lifestyle change can derail your commitment unexpectedly and easily complicate matters in many ways.

With the maintenance phase lasting the rest of your life, you have many years to continue being 'creative' and finding ways to 'motivate' yourself. As the times change, so will your situation. You may prefer swimming for exercise later on instead of pickup basketball games twice a week or jogging in the park. With the right mindset, you are going to be able to figure out what to do along the way. Certainly every chapter and all the information presented is geared to take you well into your golden years to enable you to live a healthy life and maintain a healthy weight.

For more helpful weight loss and fitness information, protocols and ideas, please subscribe to our blog at:

www.CoachJVSwann.com.